Mediterranean Small Bites

Appetizers, Snacks and Lighter Fare

By
Allyson Clarke

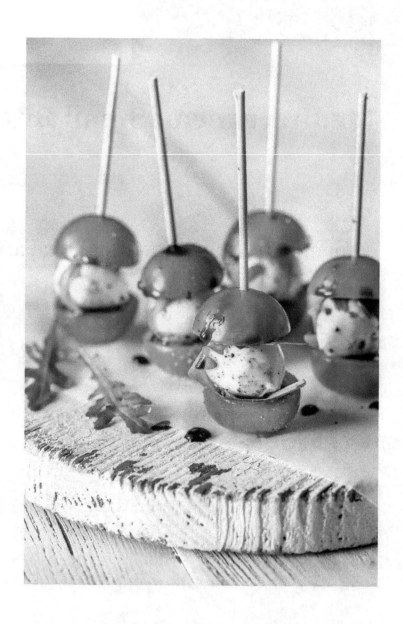

such, any inattention, use, or misuse of the information in question by the reader will render any resulting actions solely under their purview. There are no scenarios in which the publisher or the original author of this work can be in any fashion deemed liable for any hardship or damages that may befall them after undertaking information described herein.

Additionally, the information in the following pages is intended only for informational purposes and should thus be thought of as universal. As befitting its nature, it is presented without assurance regarding its prolonged validity or interim quality. Trademarks that are mentioned are done without written consent and can in no way be considered an endorsement from the trademark holder.

Table of Contents

INTRODUCTION

What is the Mediterranean Diet?

The Mediterranean diet is based on the diets of traditional eating habits from the 1960s of people from countries that surround the Mediterranean Sea, such as Greece, Italy, and Spain, and it encourages the consumption of fresh, seasonal, and local foods. The Mediterranean diet has become popular because individuals show low rates of heart disease, chronic disease, and obesity. The Mediterranean diet profile focuses on whole grains, good fats (fish, olive oil, nuts etc.), vegetables, fruits, fish, and very low consumption of any non-fish meat. Along with food, the Mediterranean diet emphasizes the need to spend time eating with family and physical activity. The Mediterranean diet is not a single prescribed diet, but rather a general food-based eating pattern, which is marked by local and cultural differences throughout the Mediterranean region.

The diet is generally characterized by a high intake of plant-based foods (e.g. fresh fruit and vegetables, nuts, and cereals) and olive oil, a moderate intake of fish and poultry, and low intakes of dairy products (mostly yoghurt and cheese), red and processed meats, and sweets. Wine is typically consumed in moderation and, normally, with a meal. A strong focus is placed on social and cultural aspects, such as communal mealtimes, resting after eating, and regular physical activity. Nowadays, however, the diet is no longer followed as widely as it was 30-50 years ago, as the diets of people living in these regions are becoming more 'Westernized' and higher in energy dense foods.

Benefits
The Mediterranean diet is not a weight loss, but increasing fiber intake and cutting out red meat, animal fats, and processed food may lead to weight loss. People who follow the diet may also have a lower risk of various diseases.

Heart health
In the 1950s,an American scientist, found that people living in the poorer areas of southern Italy had a lower risk of heart disease and death than those in wealthier parts of New York. Dr. Keys attributed this to diet. Since then, many studies have indicated that following a Mediterranean diet can help the body maintain healthy cholesterol levels and reduce the risk of high blood pressure and cardiovascular disease. The overall pattern of the Mediterranean diet is similar to their own dietary recommendations. A high proportion of calories on the diet come from fat, which can increase the risk of obesity. However, they also note that this fat is mainly unsaturated, which makes it a more healthful option than that from the typical American diet.

Protection from disease
The Mediterranean diet focuses on plant-based foods, and these are good sources of antioxidants.

The Mediterranean diet might offer protection from various cancers, and especially colorectal cancer. The reduction in risk may stem from the high intake of fruits, vegetables, and whole grains. By sticking to Mediterranean meals, people's levels of blood glucose and fats had decreased. During this time, there was also a lower incidence of stroke.

Diabetes
The Mediterranean diet may help prevent type 2 diabetes and improve markers of diabetes in people who already have the condition. Various other studies have concluded that following the Mediterranean diet can reduce the risk of type 2 diabetes and cardiovascular disease, which often occur together.

Food to eat
There is no single definition of the Mediterranean diet, but one group of scientists used the following as their 2015 basis of research.

Vegetables: Include 3 to 9 servings a day.

Fresh fruit: Up to 2 servings a day.

Cereals: Mostly whole grain from 1 to 13 servings a day.

Oil: Up to 8 servings of extra virgin (cold pressed) olive oil a day.

Fat — mostly unsaturated — made up 37% of the total calories. Unsaturated fat comes from plant sources, such as olives and avocado. The Mediterranean diet also provided 33 grams (g) of fiber a day. The baseline diet for this study provided around

2,200 calories a day. Typical ingredients. Here are some examples of ingredients that people often include in the Mediterranean diet.

Vegetables: Tomatoes, peppers, onions, eggplant, zucchini, cucumber, leafy green vegetables, plus others.

Fruits: Melon, apples, apricots, peaches, oranges, and lemons, and so on.

Legumes: Beans, lentils, and chickpeas.

Nuts and seeds: Almonds, walnuts, sunflower seeds, and cashews.

Unsaturated fat: Olive oil, sunflower oil, olives, and avocados.

Dairy products: Cheese and yogurt are the main dairy foods.

Cereals: These are mostly whole grain and include wheat and rice with bread accompanying many meals.

Fish: Sardines and other oily fish, as well as oysters and other shellfish. Poultry: Chicken or turkey.

Eggs: Chicken, quail, and duck eggs.

Drinks: A person can drink red wine in moderation.

The Mediterranean diet does not include strong liquor or carbonated and sweetened drinks. According to one definition, the diet limits red meat and sweets to less than 2 servings per week.

Food to avoid

Here's a list of foods you should generally limit while eating Mediterranean-style meals. Heavily processed foods. Let's be real: Many, many foods are processed to some degree. A can of beans has been processed, in the sense that the beans have been cooked before being canned. Olive oil has been processed, because olives have been turned into oil. But when we talk about limiting processed foods, this really means avoiding things like frozen meals with tons of sodium. You should also limit soda, desserts and candy. As the adage goes, if the ingredient list includes items that your great-grandparents wouldn't recognize as food, it's probably processed. If you're buying a packaged food that's as close to its whole-food form as possible — such as frozen fruit or veggies with nothing added — you're good to go.

Processed red meat

On the Mediterranean diet, you should minimize your intake of red meat, such as steak. What about processed red meat, such as hot dogs and bacon? You should avoid these foods or limit them as much as possible. A study published in BMJ found that regularly eating red meat, especially processed varieties, was associated with a higher risk of death. Butter. Here's another food that should be limited on the Mediterranean diet. Use olive oil instead, which has many heart health benefits and contains less saturated fat than butter. According to the USDA National Nutrient Database, butter has 7 grams of saturated fat per tablespoon, while olive oil has about 2 grams.

Refined grains

The Mediterranean diet is centered around whole grains, such as farro, millet, couscous and brown rice. With this eating style, you'll generally want to limit your intake of refined grains such as white pasta and white bread.

Alcohol

When you're following the Mediterranean diet, red wine should be your chosen alcoholic drink. This is because red wine offers health benefits, particularly for the heart. But it's important to limit intake of any type of alcohol to up to one drink per day for women, as well as men older than 65, and up to two drinks daily for men age 65 and younger. The amount that counts as a drink is 5 ounces of wine, 12 ounces of beer or 1.5 ounces of 80-proof liquor.

Parmesan Chips

Servings: 4

Cooking Time: 20 Minutes

Ingredients:

- 1 zucchini
- 2 oz Parmesan, grated
- ½ teaspoon paprika
- 1 teaspoon olive oil

Directions:

1. Trim zucchini and slice it into the chips with the help of the vegetable slices.

2. Then mix up together Parmesan and paprika.

3. Sprinkle the zucchini chips with olive oil.

4. After this, dip every zucchini slice in the cheese mixture.

5. Place the zucchini chips in the lined baking tray and bake for 20 minutes at 375F.

6. Flip the zucchini sliced onto another side after 10 minutes of cooking. 7. Chill the cooked chips well.

Nutrition Info:Per Serving:calories 64, fat 4.3, fiber 0.6, carbs 2.3, protein 5.2

Chicken Bites

Servings: 6

Cooking Time: 5 Minutes

Ingredients:

- ½ cup coconut flakes
- 8 oz chicken fillet
- ¼ cup Greek yogurt
- 1 teaspoon dried dill
- 1 teaspoon salt
- 1 teaspoon ground black pepper
- 1 tablespoon tomato sauce
- 1 teaspoon honey
- 4 tablespoons sunflower oil

Directions:

1. Chop the chicken fillet on the small cubes (popcorn cubes)
2. Sprinkle them with dried dill, salt, and ground black pepper.
3. Then add Greek yogurt and stir carefully.
4. After this, pour sunflower oil in the skillet and heat it up.

5. Coat chicken cubes in the coconut flakes and roast in the hot oil for 3-4 minutes or until the popcorn cubes are golden brown.

6. Dry the popcorn chicken with the help of the paper towel. 7. Make the sweet sauce: whisk together honey and tomato sauce. 8. Serve the popcorn chicken hot or warm with sweet sauce.

Nutrition Info:Per Serving:calories 107, fat 5.2, fiber 0.8, carbs 2.8, protein 12.1

Chicken Kale Wraps

Servings: 4

Cooking Time: 10 Minutes

Ingredients:

- 4 kale leaves
- 4 oz chicken fillet
- ½ apple
- 1 tablespoon butter
- ¼ teaspoon chili pepper
- ¾ teaspoon salt
- 1 tablespoon lemon juice
- ¾ teaspoon dried thyme

Directions:

1. Chop the chicken fillet into the small cubes.

2. Then mix up together chicken with chili pepper and salt.

3. Heat up butter in the skillet.

4. Add chicken cubes. Roast them for 4 minutes.

5. Meanwhile, chop the apple into small cubes and add it in the chicken.

6. Mix up well.

7. Sprinkle the ingredients with lemon juice and dried thyme.

8. Cook them for 5 minutes over the medium-high heat.

9. Fill the kale leaves with the hot chicken mixture and wrap.

Nutrition Info:Per Serving:calories 106, fat 5.1, fiber 1.1, carbs 6.3, protein 9

Savory Pita Chips

Servings: 1 Cup

Cooking Time: 10 Minutes

Ingredients:

- 3 pitas
- 1/4 cup extra-virgin olive oil
- 1/4 cup zaatar

Directions:

1. Preheat the oven to 450°F.
2. Cut pitas into 2-inch pieces, and place in a large bowl.
3. Drizzle pitas with extra-virgin olive oil, sprinkle with zaatar, and toss to coat.
4. Spread out pitas on a baking sheet, and bake for 8 to 10 minutes or until lightly browned and crunchy.
5. Let pita chips cool before removing from the baking sheet. Store in an airtight container for up to 1 month.

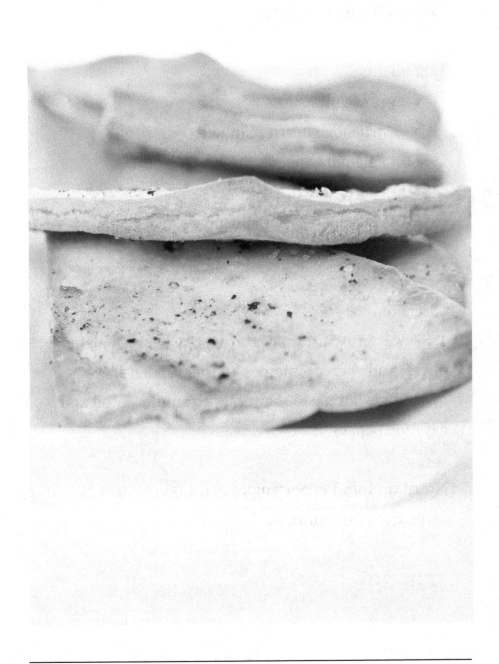

Artichoke Skewers

Servings: 4

Cooking Time: 0 Minutes

Ingredients:

- 4 prosciutto slices
- 4 artichoke hearts, canned
- 4 kalamata olives
- 4 cherry tomatoes
- ¼ teaspoon cayenne pepper
- ¼ teaspoon sunflower oil

Directions:

1. Skewer prosciutto slices, artichoke hearts, kalamata olives, and cherry tomatoes on the wooden skewers.
2. Sprinkle antipasto skewers with sunflower oil and cayenne pepper.

Nutrition Info:Per Serving:calories 152, fat 3.7, fiber 10.8, carbs 23.2, protein 11.1

Kidney Bean Spread

Servings: 4

Cooking Time: 18 Minutes

Ingredients:

- 1 lb dry kidney beans, soaked overnight and drained
- 1 tsp garlic, minced
- 2 tbsp olive oil
- 1 tbsp fresh lemon juice
- 1 tbsp paprika
- 4 cups vegetable stock
- 1/2 cup onion, chopped
- Pepper
- Salt

Directions:

1. Add beans and stock into the instant pot.

2. Seal pot with lid and cook on high for 18 minutes.

3. Once done, allow to release pressure naturally. Remove lid.

4. Drain beans well and reserve 1/2 cup stock.

5. Transfer beans, reserve stock, and remaining ingredients into the food processor and process until smooth.

6. Serve and enjoy.

Nutrition Info: Calories 461 Fat 8.6 g Carbohydrates 73 g Sugar 4 g Protein 26.4 g Cholesterol 0 mg

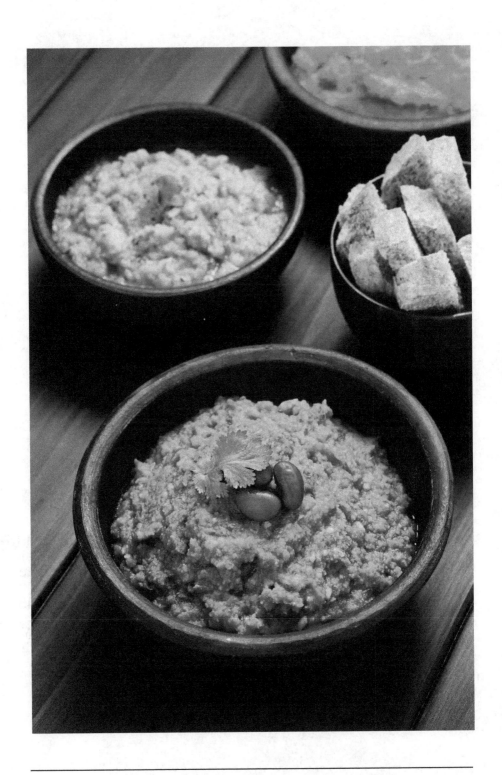

Mediterranean Polenta Cups Recipe

Servings: 24

Cooking Time: 5 Minutes

Ingredients:

- 1 cup yellow cornmeal
- 1 garlic clove, minced
- 1/2 teaspoon fresh thyme, minced or 1/4 teaspoon dried thyme 1/2 teaspoon salt
- 1/4 cup feta cheese, crumbled
- 1/4 teaspoon pepper
- 2 tablespoons fresh basil, chopped
- 4 cups water
- 4 plum tomatoes, finely chopped

Directions:

1. In a heavy, large saucepan, bring the water and the salt to a boil; reduce the heat to a gentle boil. Slowly whisk in the cornmeal; cook, stirring with a wooden spoon for about 15 to 20 minutes, or until the polenta is thick and pulls away cleanly from the sides of the pan. Remove from the heat; stir in the pepper and the thyme.

2. Grease miniature muffin cups with cooking spray. Spoon a heaping tablespoon of the polenta mixture into each muffin cups.

3. With the back of a spoon, make an indentation in the center of each; cover and chill until the mixture is set.

4. Meanwhile, combine the feta cheese, tomatoes, garlic, and basil in a small-sized bowl.

5. Unmold the chilled polenta cups; place them on an ungreased baking sheet. Tops each indentation with 1 heaping tablespoon of the feta mixture. Broil the cups 4 inches from the heat source for about 5 to 7 minutes, or until heated through.

Nutrition Info:Per Serving:26 cal, 1 mg chol., 62 mg sodium, 5 g carbs., 1 g fiber, and 1 g protein.

Tomato Triangles

Servings: 6

Cooking Time: 0 Minutes

Ingredients:

- 6 corn tortillas
- 1 tablespoon cream cheese
- 1 tablespoon ricotta cheese
- ½ teaspoon minced garlic
- 1 tablespoon fresh dill, chopped
- 2 tomatoes, sliced

Directions:

1. Cut every tortilla into 2 triangles.

2. Then mix up together cream cheese, ricotta cheese, minced garlic, and dill.

3. Spread 6 triangles with cream cheese mixture.

4. Then place sliced tomato on them and cover with remaining tortilla triangles.

Nutrition Info:Per Serving:calories 71, fat 1.6, fiber 2.1, carbs 12.8, protein 2.3

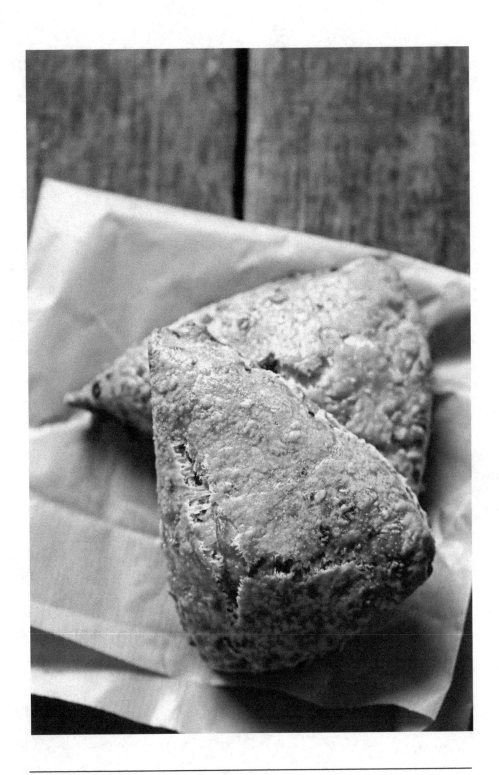

Chili Mango And Watermelon Salsa

Servings: 12

Cooking Time: 0 Minutes

Ingredients:

- 1 red tomato, chopped
- Salt and black pepper to the taste
- 1 cup watermelon, seedless, peeled and cubed
- 1 red onion, chopped
- 2 mangos, peeled and chopped
- 2 chili peppers, chopped
- ¼ cup cilantro, chopped
- 3 tablespoons lime juice
- Pita chips for serving

Directions:

1. In a bowl, mix the tomato with the watermelon, the onion and the rest of the ingredients except the pita chips and toss well.
2. Divide the mix into small cups and serve with pita chips on the side.

Nutrition Info: calories 62, fat 4.7, fiber 1.3, carbs 3.9, protein 2.3

Tomato Olive Salsa

Servings: 4

Cooking Time: 5 Minutes

Ingredients:

- 2 cups olives, pitted and chopped
- 1/4 cup fresh parsley, chopped
- 1/4 cup fresh basil, chopped
- 2 tbsp green onion, chopped
- 1 cup grape tomatoes, halved
- 1 tbsp olive oil
- 1 tbsp vinegar
- Pepper
- Salt

Directions:

1. Add all ingredients into the inner pot of instant pot and stir well.

2. Seal pot with lid and cook on high for 5 minutes.

3. Once done, allow to release pressure naturally for 5 minutes then release remaining using quick release. Remove lid.

4. Stir well and serve.

Nutrition Info: Calories 119 Fat 10.8 g Carbohydrates 6.5 g Sugar 1.3 g Protein 1.2 g Cholesterol 0 mg

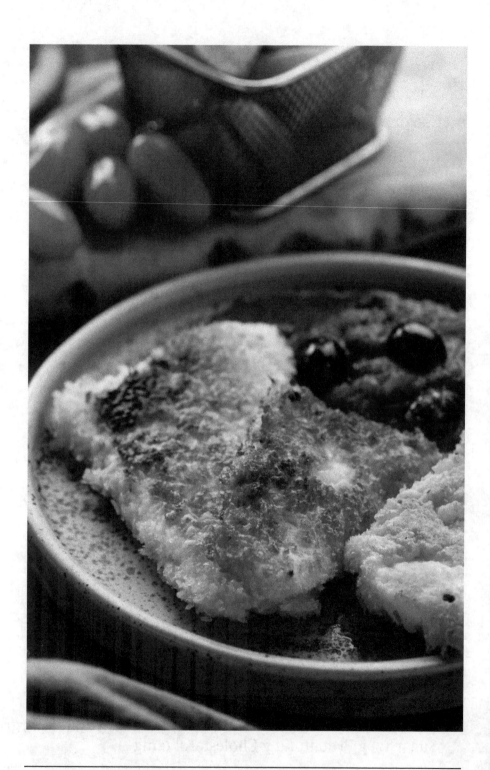

Lavash Chips

Servings: 4

Cooking Time: 10 Minutes

Ingredients:

- 1 lavash sheet, whole grain
- 1 tablespoon canola oil
- 1 teaspoon paprika
- ½ teaspoon chili pepper
- ½ teaspoon salt

Directions:

1. In the shallow bowl whisk together canola oil, paprika, chili pepper, and salt.
2. Then chop lavash sheet roughly (in the shape of chips).
3. Sprinkle lavash chips with oil mixture and arrange in the tray to get one thin layer.
4. Bake the lavash chips for 10 minutes at 365F. Flip them on another side from time to time to avoid burning.
5. Cool the cooked chips well.

Nutrition Info:Per Serving:calories 73, fat 4, fiber 0.7, carbs 8.4, protein 1.6

Homemade Salsa

Servings: 8

Cooking Time: 5 Minutes

Ingredients:

- 12 oz grape tomatoes, halved
- 1/4 cup fresh cilantro, chopped
- 1 fresh lime juice
- 28 oz tomatoes, crushed
- 1 tbsp garlic, minced
- 1 green bell pepper, chopped
- 1 red bell pepper, chopped
- 2 onions, chopped
- 6 whole tomatoes
- Salt

Directions:

1. Add whole tomatoes into the instant pot and gently smash the tomatoes.
2. Add remaining ingredients except cilantro, lime juice, and salt and stir well.
3. Seal pot with lid and cook on high for 5 minutes.

4. Once done, allow to release pressure naturally for 10 minutes then release remaining using quick release. Remove lid.

5. Add cilantro, lime juice, and salt and stir well.

6. Serve and enjoy.

Nutrition Info: Calories 146 Fat 1.2 g Carbohydrates 33.2 g Sugar 4 g Protein 6.9 g Cholesterol 0 mg

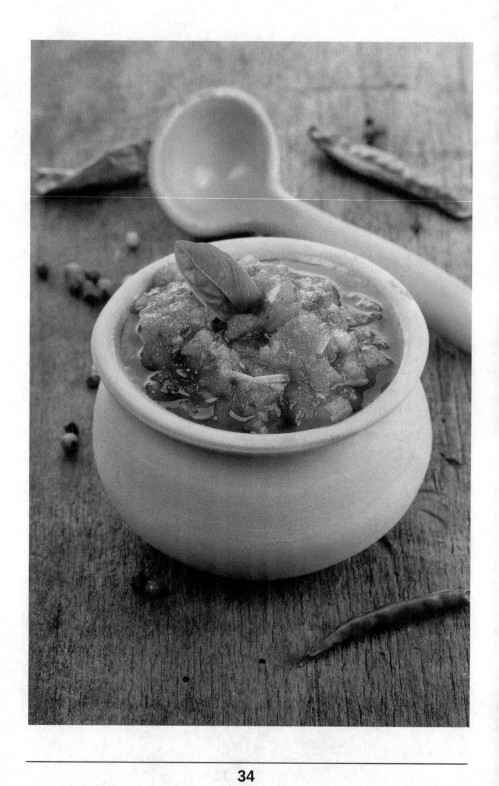

Stuffed Zucchinis

Servings: 6

Cooking Time: 40 Minutes

Ingredients:

- 6 zucchinis, halved lengthwise and insides scooped out
- 2 garlic cloves, minced
- 2 tablespoons oregano, chopped
- Juice of 2 lemons
- Salt and black pepper to the taste
- 2 tablespoons olive oil
- 8 ounces feta cheese, crumbed

Directions:

1. Arrange the zucchini halves on a baking sheet lined with parchment paper, divide the cheese and the rest of the ingredients in each zucchini half and bake at 450 degrees F for 40 minutes.

2. Arrange the stuffed zucchinis on a platter and serve as an appetizer.

Yogurt Dip

Servings: 6

Cooking Time: 0 Minutes

Ingredients:

- 2 cups Greek yogurt
- 2 tablespoons pistachios, toasted and chopped
- A pinch of salt and white pepper
- 2 tablespoons mint, chopped
- 1 tablespoon kalamata olives, pitted and chopped
- ¼ cup za'atar spice
- ¼ cup pomegranate seeds
- 1/3 cup olive oil

Directions:

1. In a bowl, combine the yogurt with the pistachios and the rest of the ingredients, whisk well, divide into small cups and serve with pita chips on the side.

Nutrition Info: calories 294, fat 18, fiber 1, carbs 21, protein 10

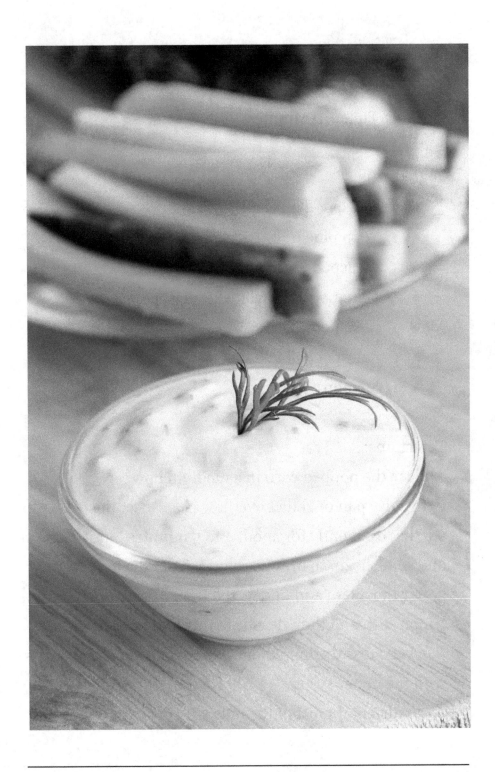

Popcorn-pine Nut Mix

Servings: 10

Cooking Time: 10 Minutes

Ingredients:

- 1 tablespoon olive oil
- 1/2 cup pine nuts
- 1/2 teaspoon Italian seasoning
- 1/4 cup popcorn, white kernels, popped
- 1/4 teaspoon salt
- 2 tablespoons honey
- 1/2 lemon zest

Directions:

1. Place the popped corn in a medium bowl.

2. In a dry pan or skillet over low heat, toast the pine nuts, stirring frequently for about 4 to 5 minutes, until fragrant and some begin to brown; remove from the heat.

3. Stir the oil in; add honey, the Italian seasoning, the lemon zest, and the salt. Stir to mix and pour over the popcorn; toss the ingredients to coat the popcorn kernels with the honey syrup.

4. It's alright if most of the nuts sink in the bowl bottom.

5. Let the mixture sit for about 2 minutes to allow the honey to cool and to get stickier.

6. Transfer the bowl contents into a Servings: bowl so the nuts are on the top. Gently stir and serve.

Nutrition Info:Per Serving:80 cal, 6 g total fat (0.5 g sat. fat), 0 mg chol., 105 mg sodium, 60 mg pot., 5 total carbs., <1 g fiber, 4 g sugar, 2 g protein, 2% vitamin A, 8% vitamin C, 4% calcium, and 4% iron.

Scallions Dip

Servings: 8

Cooking Time: 0 Minutes

Ingredients:

- 6 scallions, chopped
- 1 garlic clove, minced
- 3 tablespoons olive oil
- Salt and black pepper to the taste
- 1 tablespoon lemon juice
- 1 and ½ cups cream cheese, soft
- 2 ounces prosciutto, cooked and crumbled

Directions:

1. In a bowl, mix the scallions with the garlic and the rest of the ingredients except the prosciutto and whisk well.
2. Divide into bowls, sprinkle the prosciutto on top and serve as a party dip.

Nutrition Info: calories 144, fat 7.7, fiber 1.4, carbs 6.3, protein 5.5

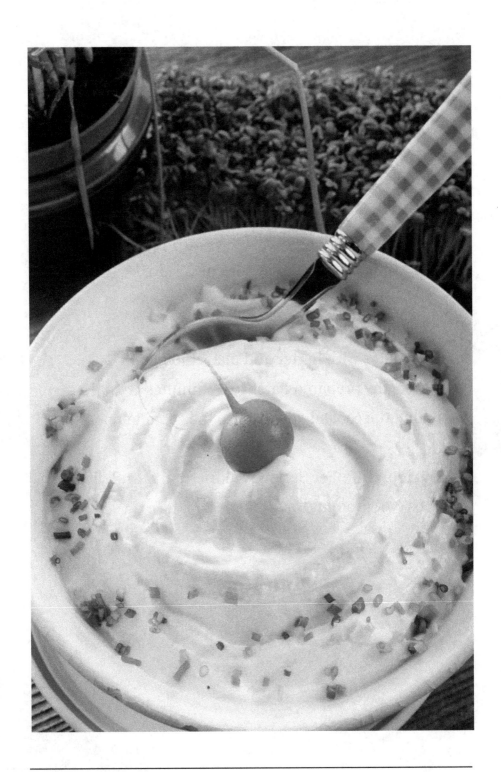

Date Balls

Servings: 3

Cooking Time: 5 Minutes

Ingredients:

- 3 dates, pitted
- 3 pistachio nuts
- ½ teaspoon butter, softened, salted

Directions:

1. Fill dates with butter and pistachio nuts.

2. Bake the prepared dates for 5 minutes at 395F.

3. Chill the cooked appetizer to the room temperature.

Nutrition Info:Per Serving:calories 42, fat 1.8, fiber 0.9, carbs 6.9, protein 0.7

Lavash Roll Ups

Servings: 2-4

Cooking Time: 10 Minutes

Ingredients:

- 2 lavash wraps (whole-wheat)
- 1/4 cup roasted red peppers, sliced
- 1/4 cup black olives, sliced
- 1/2 cup hummus of choice
- 1/2 cup grape tomatoes, halved
- 1 Medium cucumber, sliced
- Fresh dill, for garnish

Directions:

1. Lay out the lavash wraps on a clean surface. Evenly spread hummus over each piece.

2. Layer the cucumbers across the wraps, about 1/2-inch from each other, leaving about 2-icnh empty space at the bottom of the wrap for rolling purposes.

3. Place the roasted pepper slices around the cucumbers. Sprinkle with black olives and the tomatoes. Garnish with freshly chopped dill.

4. Tightly roll each wrap, using the hummus at the end to almost glue the wrap into a roll.

5. Slice each roll into 4 equal pieces. Secure each piece by sticking a toothpick through the center of each roll slice.
6. Lay each on a serving bowl or tray; garnish more with fresh dill.

Nutrition Info:Per Serving:250 cal, 8 g total fat (0.5 g sat. fat), 0 mg chol., 440 mg sodium, 340 mg pot., 43 total carbs., 40 g fiber, 3 g sugar, 10 g protein, 15% vitamin A, 25% vitamin C, 6% calcium, and 8% iron.

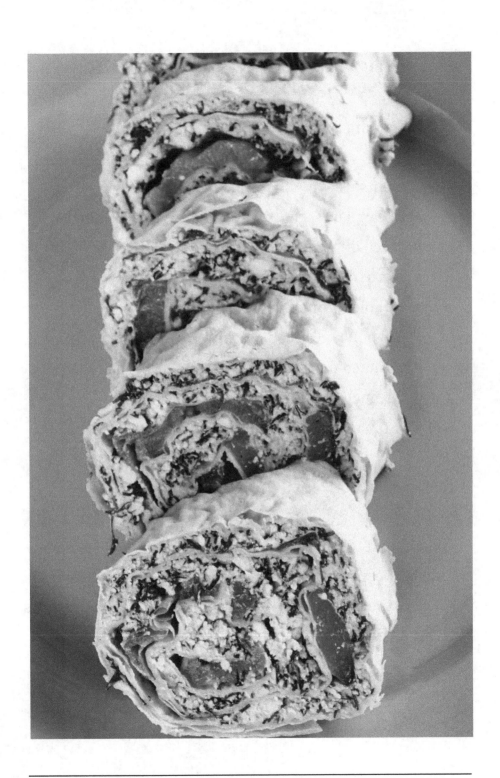

Chickpeas And Eggplant Bowls

Servings: 4

Cooking Time: 10 Minutes

Ingredients:

- 2 eggplants, cut in half lengthwise and cubed
- 1 red onion, chopped
- Juice of 1 lime
- 1 tablespoon olive oil
- 28 ounces canned chickpeas, drained and rinsed
- 1 bunch parsley, chopped
- A pinch of salt and black pepper
- 1 tablespoon balsamic vinegar

Directions:

1. Spread the eggplant cubes on a baking sheet lined with parchment paper, drizzle half of the oil all over, season with salt and pepper and cook at 425 degrees F for 10 minutes.

2. Cool the eggplant down, add the rest of the ingredients, toss, divide between appetizer plates and serve.

Nutrition Info: calories 263, fat 12, fiber 9.3, carbs 15.4, protein 7.5

Vinegar Beet Bites

Servings: 4

Cooking Time: 30 Minutes

Ingredients:

- 2 beets, sliced
- A pinch of sea salt and black pepper
- 1/3 cup balsamic vinegar
- 1 cup olive oil

Directions:

1. Spread the beet slices on a baking sheet lined with parchment paper, add the rest of the ingredients, toss and bake at 350 degrees F for 30 minutes.
2. Serve the beet bites cold as a snack.

Nutrition Info: calories 199, fat 5.4, fiber 3.5, carbs 8.5, protein 3.5

Baked Sweet-potato Fries

Servings: 6

Cooking Time: 25 Minutes

Ingredients:

- 1 1/2 teaspoons dried oregano
- 1 teaspoon dried thyme
- 1 teaspoon garlic powder
- 1/2 teaspoon salt
- 2 large sweet potatoes (about 2 pounds), skins on, scrubbed, cut into 1/2-inch thick 4-inch long sticks
- 3 large egg whites (a scant 1/2 cup)
- Vegetable oil, for the parchment
- For the Mediterranean spice:
- Oregano
- Thyme
- Garlic

Directions:

1. Place all of the Mediterranean spice ingredients in a small food processor or a spice grinder; briefly grind or process to blend.

2. Place the oven racks in the middle and upper position; preheat the oven to 450F.

3. Line 2 baking sheets with parchment paper; rub the paper with the oil.

4. Put the potatoes in a microwavable container, cover, and microwave for 2 minutes. Stir gently, cover, and microwave for about 1-2 minutes more or until the pieces are pliable; let rest for about 5 minutes covered. Pour into a platter.

5. In a large-sized bowl, whisk the eggs until frothy. Add the spice mix and whisk again to blend.

6. Working in batches, toss the sweet potatoes in the seasoned egg whites letting the excess liquid drip back into the bowl. Arrange the coated potatoes in a single layer on the prepared baking sheets.

7. Bake for 10 minutes; flip the pieces over using a spatula. Rotate the baking sheets from back to front and one to the other; bake for about 15 minutes or until dark golden brown. Serve immediately.

Nutrition Info:Per Serving:100 cal., 4 g total fat (0 g sat. fat), 0 mg chol., 60 mg sodium, 230 mg pot., 12 g total carbs., 2 g fiber, 2 g sugar, 3 g protein, 150% vitamin A, 2% vitamin C, 4% calcium, and 6% iron.

Cucumber Rolls

Servings: 6

Cooking Time: 0 Minutes

Ingredients:

- 1 big cucumber, sliced lengthwise
- 1 tablespoon parsley, chopped
- 8 ounces canned tuna, drained and mashed
- Salt and black pepper to the taste
- 1 teaspoon lime juice

Directions:

1. Arrange cucumber slices on a working surface, divide the rest of the ingredients, and roll.
2. Arrange all the rolls on a platter and serve as an appetizer.

Nutrition Info: calories 200, fat 6, fiber 3.4, carbs 7.6, protein 3.5

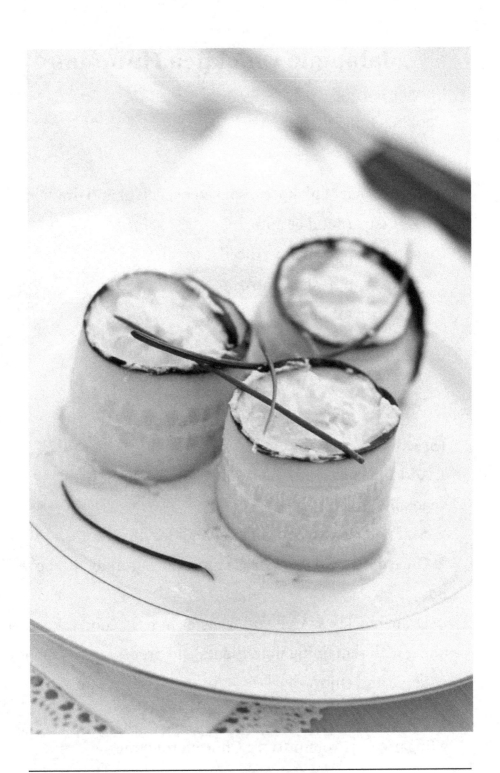

Jalapeno Chickpea Hummus

Servings: 4

Cooking Time: 25 Minutes

Ingredients:

- 1 cup dry chickpeas, soaked overnight and drained
- 1 tsp ground cumin
- 1/4 cup jalapenos, diced
- 1/2 cup fresh cilantro
- 1 tbsp tahini
- 1/2 cup olive oil
- Pepper
- Salt

Directions:

1. Add chickpeas into the instant pot and cover with vegetable stock.

2. Seal pot with lid and cook on high for 25 minutes.

3. Once done, allow to release pressure naturally. Remove lid.

4. Drain chickpeas well and transfer into the food processor along with remaining ingredients and process until smooth.

5. Serve and enjoy.

Nutrition Info: Calories 425 Fat 30.4 g Carbohydrates 31.8 g Sugar 5.6 g Protein 10.5 g Cholesterol 0 mg

Healthy Spinach Dip

Servings: 4

Cooking Time: 8 Minutes

Ingredients:

- 14 oz spinach
- 2 tbsp fresh lime juice
- 1 tbsp garlic, minced
- 2 tbsp olive oil
- 2 tbsp coconut cream
- Pepper
- Salt

Directions:

1. Add all ingredients except coconut cream into the instant pot and stir well.

2. Seal pot with lid and cook on low pressure for 8 minutes.

3. Once done, allow to release pressure naturally for 5 minutes then release remaining using quick release. Remove lid.

4. Add coconut cream and stir well and blend spinach mixture using a blender until smooth.

5. Serve and enjoy.

Nutrition Info: Calories 109 Fat 9.2 g Carbohydrates 6.6 g Sugar 1.1 g Protein 3.2 g Cholesterol 0 mg

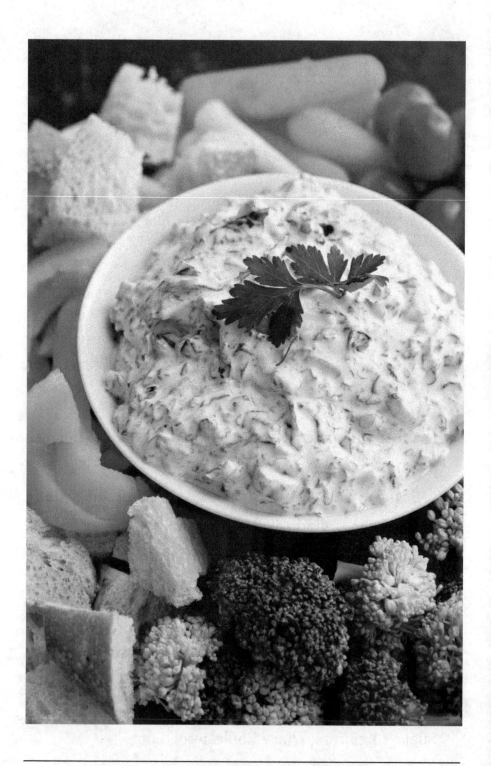

Marinated Cheese

Servings: 18

Cooking Time: 10 Minutes

Ingredients:

- 8 ounces cream cheese
- 6 sprigs fresh thyme
- 3 sprigs fresh rosemary
- 2 garlic cloves, sliced
- 1/2 cup sun-dried tomato vinaigrette dressing
- 1 teaspoon black pepper
- 1 lemon peel, cut into thin strips

Directions:

1. Cut the cream cheese into 36 cubes. Place on a serving tray.

2. Combine the remaining ingredients together.

3. Pour the dressing over the cheese; toss lightly.

4. Refrigerate for at least 1 hour to marinate.

Nutrition Info:Per Serving:44 cal., 4.3 g total fat (2.4 sat. fat), 13.9 mg chol., 40.6 mg sodium, 0.7 g total carbs., 0 g fiber, 0.4 g sugar, and 0.8 g protein.

Za'atar Fries

Servings: 5

Cooking Time: 35 Minutes

Ingredients:

- 1 teaspoon Za'atar spices
- 3 sweet potatoes
- 1 tablespoon dried dill
- 1 teaspoon salt
- 3 teaspoons sunflower oil
- ½ teaspoon paprika

Directions:

1. Pour water in the crockpot. Peel the sweet potatoes and cut them into the fries.
2. Line the baking tray with parchment.
3. Place the layer of the sweet potato in the tray.
4. Sprinkle the vegetables with dried dill, salt, and paprika.
5. Then sprinkle sweet potatoes with Za'atar and mix up well with the help of the fingertips.
6. Sprinkle the sweet potato fries with sunflower oil.
7. Preheat the oven to 375F.

8. Bake the sweet potato fries for 35 minutes. Stir the fries every 10 minutes.

Nutrition Info:Per Serving:calories 28, fat 2.9, fiber 0.2, carbs 0.6, protein 0.2

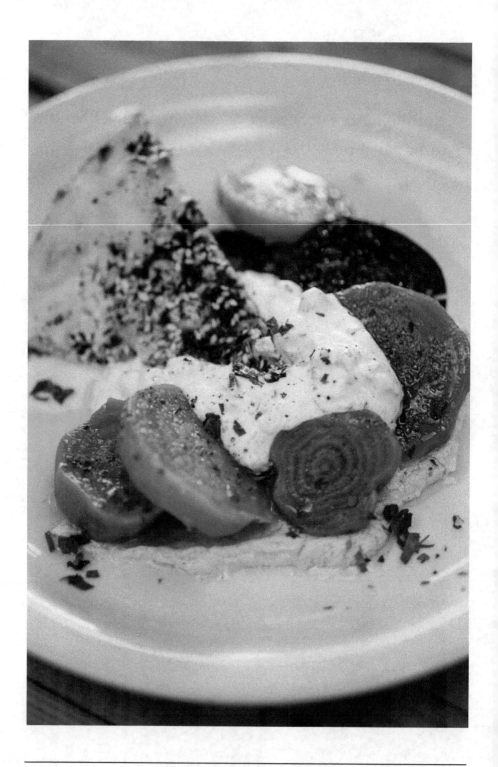

Tuna Salad

Servings: 2-4

Cooking Time: 10 Minutes

Ingredients:

- 1 can (5 ounce) albacore tuna, solid white
- 1 to 2 tablespoons mayo or Greek yogurt
- 1 whole-wheat crackers (I used sleeve Ritz®)
- 1/4 cup chickpeas, rinsed, drained (or preferred white beans)
- 1/4 cup Kalamata olives, quartered
- 1/4 cup roughly chopped marinated artichoke hearts

Directions:

1. Flake the tuna out of the can into medium-sized bowl.

2. Add the chickpeas, olives, and artichoke hearts; toss to combine.

3. Add mayo or Greek yogurt according to your taste; stir until well
combined.

4. Spoon the salad mixture onto crackers; serve.

Nutrition Info:Per Serving:130 cal., 5 g total fat (0.5 g sat. fat), 25 mg chol., 240 mg sodium, 240 mg pot., 8 g total carbs., 1 g fiber, <1 g sugar, 12 g protein, 2% vitamin A, 2% vitamin C, 4% calcium, and 6% iron.

Cheese Rolls

Servings: 1 Roll

Cooking Time: 5 Minutes

Ingredients:

- 1 cup akawi cheese
- 1 cup shredded mozzarella cheese
- 2 TB. fresh parsley, finely chopped
- 1 large egg
- 1/2 tsp. ground black pepper
- 1 large egg yolk, beaten
- 2 TB. water
- 1 pkg. egg roll dough (20 count)
- 4 TB. extra-virgin olive oil

Directions:

1. In a large bowl, combine ackawi cheese, mozzarella cheese, parsley, egg, and black pepper.

2. In a small bowl, whisk together egg yolk and water.

3. Lay out 1 egg roll, place 2 tablespoons cheese mixture at one corner of egg roll, and brush opposite corner with egg yolk mixture.

4. Fold over side of egg roll, with cheese, to the middle. Fold in left and right sides, and complete rolling egg roll,

using egg-brushed side to seal. Set aside, seal side down, and repeat with remaining egg rolls and cheese mixture.

5. In a skillet over low heat, heat 2 tablespoons extra-virgin olive oil. Add up to 4 cheese rolls, seal side down, and cook for 1 or 2 minutes per side or until browned. Repeat with remaining 2 tablespoons extra-virgin olive oil and egg rolls.

6. Serve warm.

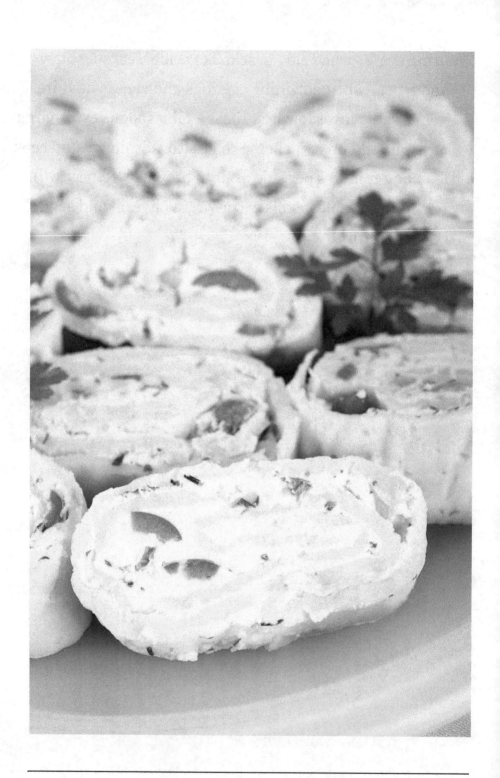

Olive, Pepperoni, And Mozzarella Bites

Servings: 2

Cooking Time: 10 Minutes

Ingredients:

- 1 pound block Mozzarella cheese
- 1 package pepperoni
- 1 can whole medium black olives

Directions:

1. Slice the block of mozzarella cheese into 1/2x1/2-inch cubes. Drain the olives from the liquid.

2. With a toothpick, skewer the olive, pushing it 1/3 way up the toothpick.

3. Fold a pepperoni into half or quarters and skewer after the olive.

4. Finally, skewer a mozzarella cheese, not pushing all the way through the cube, about only half way through. Repeat with the remaining olives, pepperoni, and mozzarella cubes.

Nutrition Info:Per Serving:75 cal., 5.6 g total fat (2.5 g sat. fat), 14 mg chol., 221 mg sodium, 16 mg pot., 0.8 g total carbs., 0 g fiber, 0 g sugar, 5.6 g protein, 3% vitamin A, 0% vitamin C, 11% calcium, and 1% iron.

Eggplant Dip

Servings: 4

Cooking Time: 40 Minutes

Ingredients:

- 1 eggplant, poked with a fork
- 2 tablespoons tahini paste
- 2 tablespoons lemon juice
- 2 garlic cloves, minced
- 1 tablespoon olive oil
- Salt and black pepper to the taste
- 1 tablespoon parsley, chopped

Directions:

1. Put the eggplant in a roasting pan, bake at 400 degrees F for 40 minutes, cool down, peel and transfer to your food processor.

2. Add the rest of the ingredients except the parsley, pulse well, divide into small bowls and serve as an appetizer with the parsley sprinkled on top.

Nutrition Info: calories 121, fat 4.3, fiber 1, carbs 1.4, protein 4.3

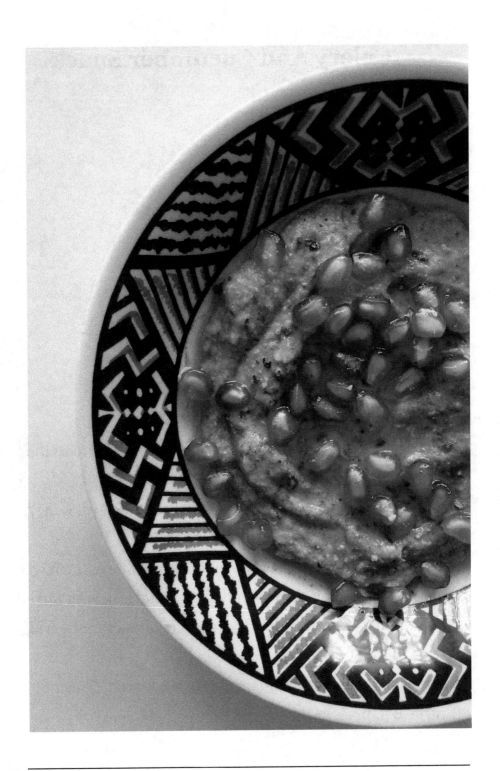

Celery And Cucumber Snack

Servings: 4

Cooking Time: 0 Minutes

Ingredients:

- 6 oz celery stalk, roughly chopped
- 2 cucumbers, roughly chopped
- 1 teaspoon mustard
- 1 teaspoon honey
- 2 teaspoons lemon juice
- 1 tablespoon fresh cilantro, chopped

Directions:

1. Place celery stalk, cucumbers, and fresh cilantro in the big bowl.

2. In the shallow bowl combine together mustard, honey, and lemon juice.

3. Pour the liquid over the vegetables and shake them well.

4. Transfer the vegetables in the jars and close with the lid.

5. Store the vegetable snack jars up to 2 hours in the fridge.

Nutrition Info:Per Serving:calories 39, fat 0.5, fiber 1.6, carbs 8.5, protein 1.5

Oat Bites

Servings: 4

Cooking Time: 10 Minutes

Ingredients:

- 1 teaspoon honey
- 4 dates, pitted
- 1 tablespoon rolled oats
- 1 tablespoon raisins, chopped
- ¼ teaspoon ground cinnamon
- 1 teaspoon chia seeds, dried

Directions:

1. Mash the dates with the help of the fork until you get a mashed mixture.

2. Then add honey, rolled oats, raisins, ground cinnamon, and chia seeds.

3. Mix up the mixture with the help of the spoon until homogenous.

4. Make the small balls and refrigerate them for at least 10-15 minutes.

Nutrition Info:Per Serving:calories 52, fat 0.9, fiber 1.8, carbs 11.4, protein 0.9

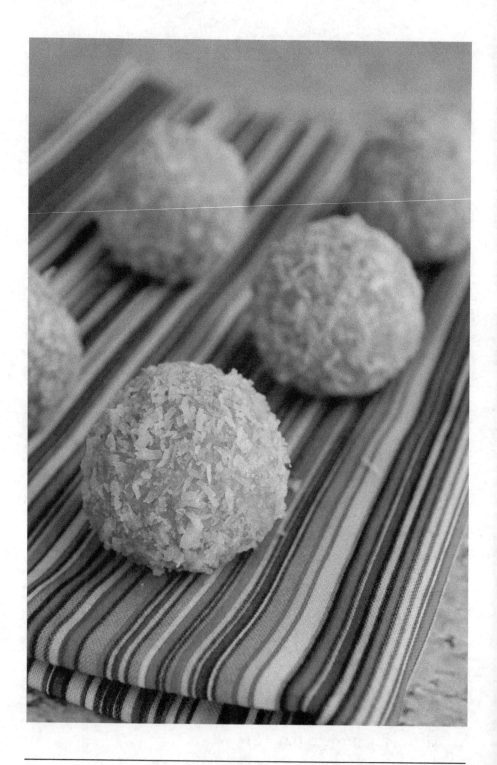

Eggplant Bites

Servings: 8

Cooking Time: 15 Minutes

Ingredients:
- 2 eggplants, cut into 20 slices
- 2 tablespoons olive oil
- ½ cup roasted peppers, chopped
- ½ cup kalamata olives, pitted and chopped
- 1 tablespoon lime juice
- 1 teaspoon red pepper flakes, crushed
- Salt and black pepper to the taste
- 2 tablespoons mint, chopped

Directions:

1. In a bowl, mix the roasted peppers with the olives, half of the oil and the rest of the ingredients except the eggplant slices and stir well.

2. Brush eggplant slices with the rest of the olive oil on both sides, place them on the preheated grill over medium high heat, cook for 7 minutes on each side and transfer them to a platter.

3. Top each eggplant slice with roasted peppers mix and serve.

Nutrition Info: calories 214, fat 10.6, fiber 5.8, carbs 15.4, protein 5.4

Creamy Pepper Spread

Servings: 4

Cooking Time: 15 Minutes

Ingredients:

- 1 lb red bell peppers, chopped and remove seeds
- 1 1/2 tbsp fresh basil
- 1 tbsp olive oil
- 1 tbsp fresh lime juice
- 1 tsp garlic, minced
- Pepper
- Salt

Directions:

1. Add all ingredients into the inner pot of instant pot and stir well.

2. Seal pot with lid and cook on high for 15 minutes.

3. Once done, allow to release pressure naturally for 10 minutes then release remaining using quick release. Remove lid.

4. Transfer bell pepper mixture into the food processor and process until smooth.

5. Serve and enjoy.

Nutrition Info: Calories 41 Fat 3.6 g Carbohydrates 3.5 g Sugar 1.7 g Protein 0.4 g Cholesterol 0 mg

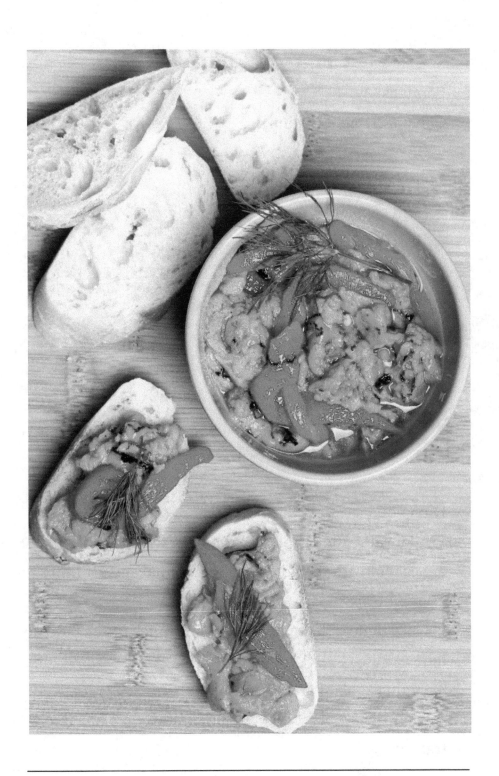

Creamy Eggplant Dip

Servings: 4

Cooking Time: 20 Minutes

Ingredients:
- 1 eggplant
- 1/2 tsp paprika
- 1 tbsp olive oil
- 1 tbsp fresh lime juice
- 2 tbsp tahini
- 1 garlic clove
- 1 cup of water
- Pepper
- Salt

Directions:

1. Add water and eggplant into the instant pot.

2. Seal pot with the lid and select manual and set timer for 20 minutes.

3. Once done, release pressure using quick release. Remove lid.

4. Drain eggplant and let it cool.

5. Once the eggplant is cool then remove eggplant skin and transfer

eggplant flesh into the food processor.

6. Add remaining ingredients into the food processor and process until smooth.

7. Serve and enjoy.

Nutrition Info: Calories 108 Fat 7.8 g Carbohydrates 9.7 g Sugar 3.7 g Protein 2.5 g Cholesterol 0 mg

Herbed Goat Cheese Dip

Servings: 4

Cooking Time: 0 Minutes

Ingredients:

- ¼ cup mixed parsley, chopped
- ¼ cup chives, chopped
- 8 ounces goat cheese, soft
- Salt and black pepper to the taste
- A drizzle of olive oil

Directions:

1. In your food processor mix the goat cheese with the parsley and the rest of the ingredients and pulse well.
2. Divide into small bowls and serve as a party dip.

Nutrition Info: calories 245, fat 11.3, fiber 4.5, carbs 8.9, protein 11.2

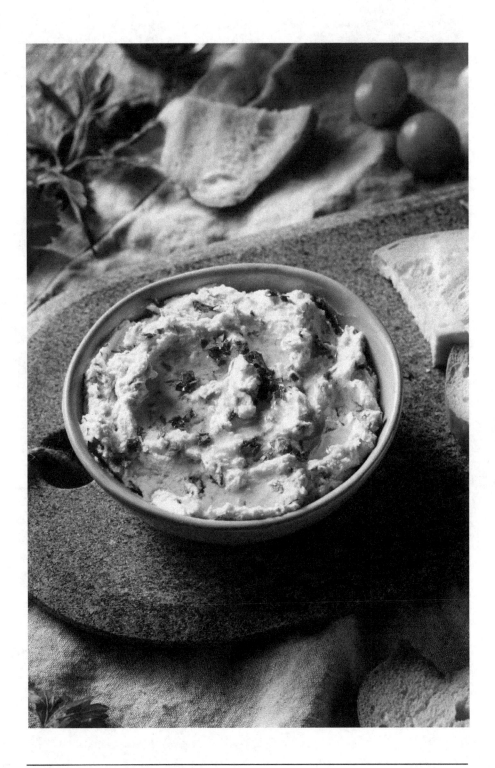

Italian Wheatberry Cakes

Servings: 6

Cooking Time: 15 Minutes

Ingredients:

- 1 cup wheatberry, cooked
- 2 eggs
- ¼ cup ground chicken
- 1 tablespoon wheat flour, whole grain
- 1 teaspoon Italian seasoning
- 1 tablespoon olive oil
- 1 teaspoon salt

Directions:

1. In the mixing bowl mix up together wheatberry and ground chicken.

2. Crack eggs in the mixture.

3. Then add wheat flour, Italian seasoning, and salt.

4. Mix up the mass with the help of the spoon until homogenous.

5. Then make burgers and freeze them in the freezer for 20 minutes.

6. Heat up olive oil in the skillet.

7. Place frozen burgers in the hot oil and roast them for 4 minutes from each side over the high heat.

8. Then cook burgers for 10 minutes more over the medium heat. Flip them onto another side from time to time.

Nutrition Info:Per Serving:calories 97, fat 5.7, fiber 1.5, carbs 9.2, protein 5.2

Healthy Kidney Bean Dip

Servings: 6

Cooking Time: 10 Minutes

Ingredients:

- 1 cup dry white kidney beans, soaked overnight and drained
- 1 tbsp fresh lemon juice
- 2 tbsp water
- 1/2 cup coconut yogurt
- 1 roasted garlic clove
- 1 tbsp olive oil
- 1/4 tsp cayenne
- 1 tsp dried parsley
- Pepper
- Salt

Directions:

1. Add soaked beans and 1 3/4 cups of water into the instant pot.

2. Seal pot with lid and cook on high for 10 minutes.

3. Once done, allow to release pressure naturally. Remove lid.

4. Drain beans well and transfer them into the food processor.

5. Add remaining ingredients into the food processor and process until smooth.

6. Serve and enjoy.

Nutrition Info: Calories 136 Fat 3.2 g Carbohydrates 20 g Sugar 2.1 g Protein 7.7 g Cholesterol 0 mg

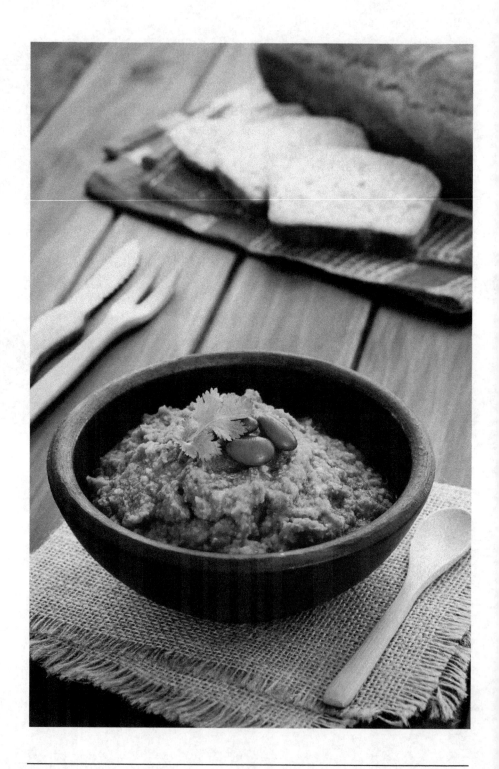

Lentils Spread

Servings: 12

Cooking Time: 0 Minutes

Ingredients:

- 1 garlic clove, minced
- 12 ounces canned lentils, drained and rinsed
- 1 teaspoon oregano, dried
- ¼ teaspoon basil, dried
- 3 tablespoons olive oil
- 1 tablespoon balsamic vinegar
- Salt and black pepper to the taste

Directions:

1. In a blender, combine the lentils with the garlic and the rest of the ingredients, pulse well, divide into bowls and serve as an appetizer

.

Nutrition Info: calories 287, fat 9.5, fiber 3.5, carbs 15.3, protein 9.3

Chickpeas Spread

Servings: 7

Cooking Time: 45 Minutes

Ingredients:

- 1 cup chickpeas, soaked
- 6 cups of water
- ½ cup lemon juice
- 3 tablespoon olive oil
- 1 teaspoon salt
- 1/3 teaspoon harissa

Directions:

1. Combine together chickpeas and water and boil for 45 minutes or until chickpeas are tender.
2. Then transfer chickpeas in the food processor.
3. Add 1 cup of chickpeas water and lemon juice.
4. After this, add salt and harissa.
5. Blend the hummus until it is smooth and fluffy.
6. Add olive oil and pulse it for 10 seconds more.
7. Transfer the cooked hummus in the bowl and store it in the fridge up to 2 days.

Nutrition Info:Per Serving:calories 160, fat 7.9, fiber 5. carbs 17.8, protein 5.7

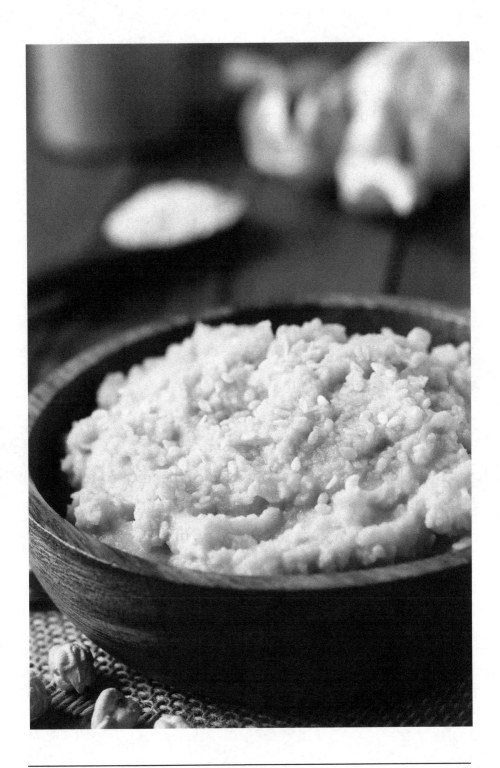

Lime Yogurt Dip

Servings: 4

Cooking Time: 0 Minutes

Ingredients:

- 1 large cucumber, trimmed
- 3 oz Greek yogurt
- 1 teaspoon olive oil
- 3 tablespoons fresh dill, chopped
- 1 tablespoon lime juice
- ¾ teaspoon salt
- 1 garlic clove, minced

Directions:

1. Grate the cucumber and squeeze the juice from it.

2. Then place the squeezed cucumber in the bowl.

3. Add Greek yogurt, olive oil, dill, lime juice, salt, and minced garlic.

4. Mix up the mixture until homogenous.

5. Store tzatziki in the fridge up to 2 days.

Nutrition Info:Per Serving:calories 44, fat 1.8, fiber 0.7, carbs 5.1, protein 3.2

Almond Bowls

Servings: 5

Cooking Time: 15 Minutes

Ingredients:

- 1 cup almonds
- 3 tablespoons salt
- 2 cups of water

Directions:

1. Bring water to boil.

2. After this, add 2 tablespoons of salt in water and stir it.

3. When salt is dissolved, add almonds and let them soak for at least 1 hour.

4. Meanwhile, line the tray with baking paper and preheat oven to 350F

5. Dry the soaked almonds with a paper towel well and arrange them in one layer in the tray.

6. Sprinkle buts with remaining salt.

7. Bake the snack for 15 minutes. Mix it from time to time with the help of the spatula or spoon.

Nutrition Info:Per Serving:calories 110, fat 9.5, fiber 2.4, carbs 4.1, protein

Beet Spread

Servings: 4

Cooking Time: 35 Minutes

Ingredients:

- 1 tablespoon pumpkin puree
- 1 beet, peeled
- 1 teaspoon tahini paste
- ½ teaspoon sesame seeds
- 1 teaspoon paprika
- 1 tablespoon olive oil
- ¼ cup water, boiled
- 1 tablespoon lime juice
- ½ teaspoon salt

Directions:

1. Place beet in the oven and bake it at 375F for 35 minutes.

2. Then chop it roughly and put in the food processor.

3. Blend the beet until smooth.

4. After this, add tahini paste, pumpkin puree, paprika, olive oil, water, lime juice, and salt.

5. Blend the hummus until smooth and fluffy.

6. Then transfer the appetizer in the bowl and sprinkle with sesame seeds.

Nutrition Info:Per Serving:calories 99, fat 8.6, fiber 1.6, carbs 3.9, protein 2.1

Calamari Mediterranean

Servings: 2

Cooking Time: 10 Minutes

Ingredients:

- 1 tablespoon Italian parsley
- 1 teaspoon ancho chili, chopped
- 1 teaspoon cumin
- 1 teaspoon red pepper flakes
- 1/2 cup white wine
- 2 cups calamari
- 2 medium plum tomatoes, diced
- 2 tablespoons capers
- 2 tablespoons garlic cloves, roasted
- 2 tablespoons olive oil
- 2 tablespoons unsalted butter
- 3 tablespoons lime juice
- Salt

Directions:

1. Heat a sauté pan. Add the oil, garlic, and the calamari; sauté for 1 minute. Add the capers, red pepper flakes, cumin, ancho chili and the diced tomatoes; cook for 1 minute.

2. Add the wine and the lime juice; simmer for 4 minutes.

3. Stir in the butter, parsley, and the salt; continue cooking until the sauce is thick.

4. Serve with whole-wheat French bread.

Nutrition Info:Per Serving:308.8 cal., 25.7 g total fat (9.3 sat. fat), 30.5 mg chol., 267.8 mg sodium, 10.2 g total carbs., 1.7 g fiber, 2.8 g sugar, and 1.9 g protein.

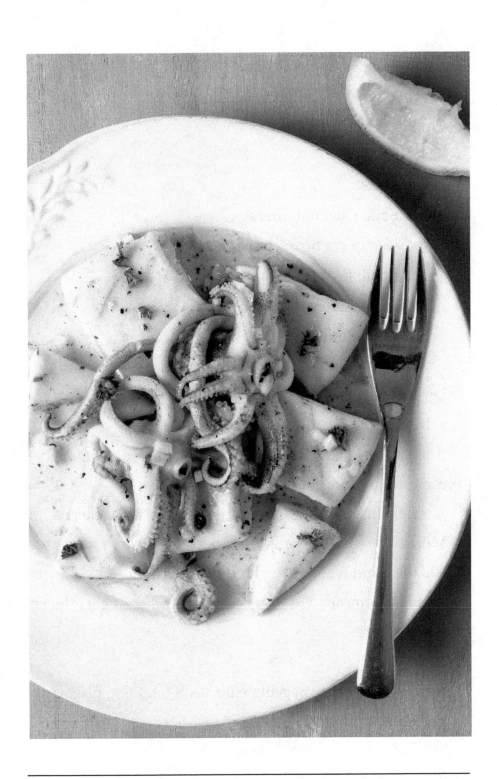

Cheddar Dip

Servings: 6

Cooking Time: 10 Minutes

Ingredients:

- 1 cup Cheddar cheese
- ¼ cup cilantro, chopped
- 1 chili pepper, chopped
- 1 teaspoon garlic powder
- ¼ cup milk

Directions:

1. Bring the milk to boil.

2. Then add Cheddar cheese in the milk and simmer the mixture for 2 minutes. Stir it constantly.

3. After this, add cilantro, chili pepper, and garlic powder. Mix up the mixture well. If it doesn't get a smooth texture, use the hand blender to blend the mass.

4. It is recommended to serve the dip when it gets the room temperature

.

Nutrition Info:Per Serving:calories 83, fat 6.5, fiber 0.1, carbs 1.2, protein 5.1

Olives And Cheese Stuffed Tomatoes

Servings: 24

Cooking Time: 0 Minutes

Ingredients:

- 24 cherry tomatoes, top cut off and insides scooped out
- 2 tablespoons olive oil
- ¼ teaspoon red pepper flakes
- ½ cup feta cheese, crumbled
- 2 tablespoons black olive paste
- ¼ cup mint, torn

Directions:

1. In a bowl, mix the olives paste with the rest of the ingredients except the cherry tomatoes and whisk well.

2. Stuff the cherry tomatoes with this mix, arrange them all on a platter and serve as an appetizer.

Nutrition Info: calories 136, fat 8.6, fiber 4.8, carbs 5.6, protein 5.1

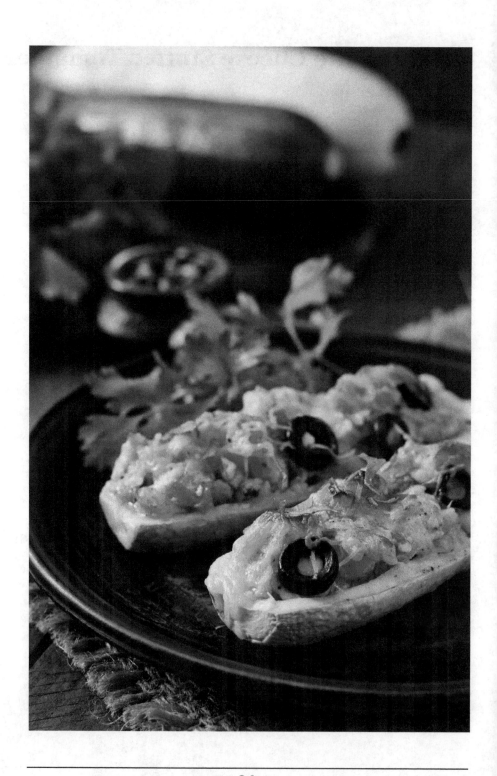

Feta Cheese Log With Sun-dried Tomatoes And Kalamata Olives

Servings: 2

Cooking Time: 20 Minutes

Ingredients:

- 8 ounces feta cheese, crumbled
- 4 ounces cream cheese, softened
- 2 tablespoons extra-virgin olive oil
- 1/8-1/4 teaspoon cayenne pepper (depending on your taste)
- 1/4 cup chopped sun-dried tomato
- 1/4 cup chopped Kalamata olive
- 1/2 teaspoon dried Mediterranean oregano, crumbled
- 1 small garlic clove, minced
- 1/2 cup walnuts, toasted, chopped
- 1/4 cup fresh parsley, minced

Directions:

1. With a mixer, combine the feta cheese, cream cheese, and the olive oil on medium speed until well combined. Add the remaining ingredients and mix well.

2. Shape the soft mixture into a 10-inch long log.

3. Combine the parsley and the walnuts; roll the log over the mixture, pressing slightly to stick the parsley and the walnuts on the sides of the log.

4. Wrap the log with plastic wrap; refrigerate for at least 5 hours to let the flavors blend.

5. Remove the plastic wrap, lay the log on a parsley-lined serving platter. Serve with whole-wheat crackers and toasted whole-wheat slices of baguette.

Nutrition Info:Per Serving:1154 cal., 106.3 g total fat (43.9 sat. fat), 226.2 mg chol., 2395.3 mg sodium, 23 g total carbs., 5 g fiber, 13.5 g sugar, and 35.2 g protein.

Lemon Salmon Rolls

Servings: 6

Cooking Time: 0 Minutes

Ingredients:

- 6 wonton wrappers
- 7 oz salmon, grilled
- 6 lettuce leaves
- 1 carrot, peeled
- 1 cucumber, trimmed
- 1 tablespoon lemon juice
- 1 teaspoon olive oil
- ¼ teaspoon dried oregano

Directions:

1. Cut the carrot and cucumber onto the wedges.

2. Then chop the grilled salmon.

3. Arrange the salmon, carrot and cucumber wedges, and lettuce leaves on 6 wonton wraps.

4. In the shallow bowl whisk together dried oregano, olive oil, and lemon juice.

5. Sprinkle the roll mixture with oil dressing and wrap.

Nutrition Info:Per Serving:calories 90, fat 3.4, fiber 0.7, carbs 7.7, protein 7.7

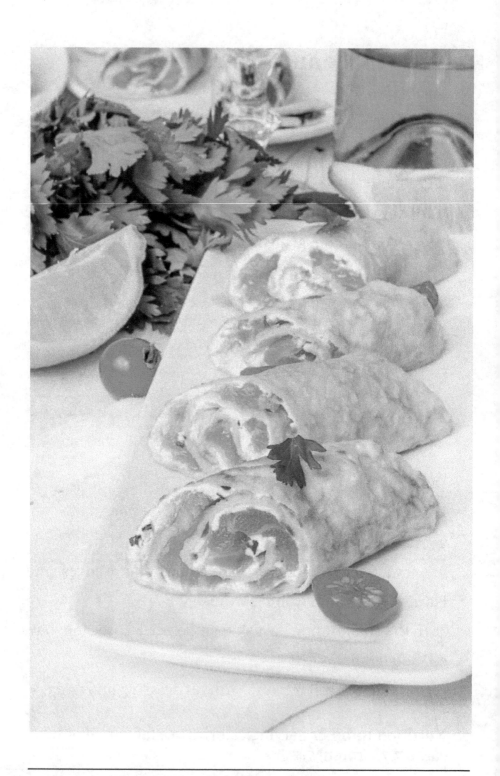

Ginger And Cream Cheese Dip

Servings: 6

Cooking Time: 0 Minutes

Ingredients:

- ½ cup ginger, grated
- 2 bunches cilantro, chopped
- 3 tablespoons balsamic vinegar
- ½ cup olive oil
- 1 and ½ cups cream cheese, soft

Directions:

1. In your blender, mix the ginger with the rest of the ingredients and pulse well.
2. Divide into small bowls and serve as a party dip.

Nutrition Info: calories 213, fat 4.9, fiber 4.1, carbs 8.8, protein 17.8

Lemon Endive Bites

Servings: 10

Cooking Time: 0 Minutes

Ingredients:

- 6 oz endive
- 2 pears, chopped
- 4 oz Blue cheese, crumbled
- 1 teaspoon olive oil
- 1 teaspoon lemon juice
- ¾ teaspoon ground cinnamon

Directions:

1. Separate endive into the spears (10 spears).

2. In the bowl combine together chopped pears, olive oil, lemon juice, ground cinnamon, and Blue cheese.

3. Fill the endive spears with cheese mixture.

Nutrition Info:Per Serving:calories 72, fat 3.8, fiber 1.9, carbs 7.4, protein 2.82.

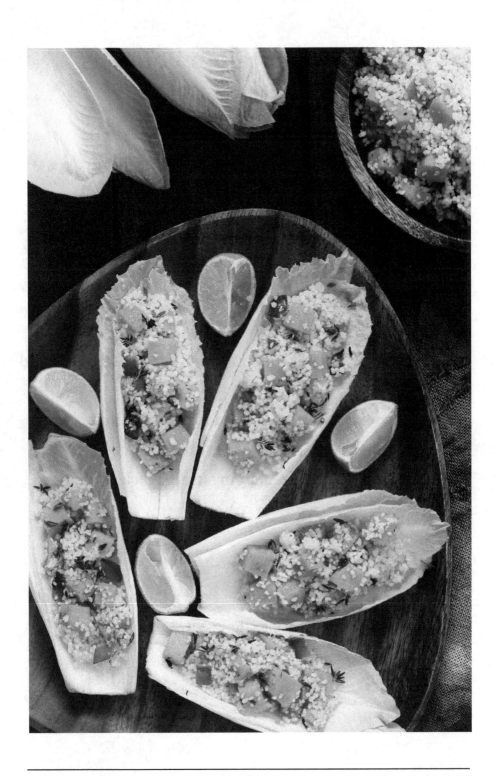

Perfect Italian Potatoes

Servings: 6

Cooking Time: 7 Minutes

Ingredients:

- 2 lbs baby potatoes, clean and cut in half
- 3/4 cup vegetable broth
- 6 oz Italian dry dressing mix

Directions:

1. Add all ingredients into the inner pot of instant pot and stir well
2. Seal pot with lid and cook on high for 7 minutes.
3. Once done, allow to release pressure naturally for 3 minutes then release remaining using quick release. Remove lid.
4. Stir well and serve.

Nutrition Info: Calories 149 Fat 0.3 g Carbohydrates 41.6 g Sugar 11.4 g Protein 4.5 g Cholesterol 0 mg

Feta Artichoke Dip

Servings: 8

Cooking Time: 30 Minutes

Ingredients:

- 8 ounces artichoke hearts, drained and quartered
- ¾ cup basil, chopped
- ¾ cup green olives, pitted and chopped
- 1 cup parmesan cheese, grated
- 5 ounces feta cheese, crumbled

Directions:

1. In your food processor, mix the artichokes with the basil and the rest of the ingredients, pulse well, and transfer to a baking dish.

2. Introduce in the oven, bake at 375 degrees F for 30 minutes and serve as a party dip.

Nutrition Info: calories 186, fat 12.4, fiber 0.9, carbs 2.6, protein 1.5

Peach Skewers

Servings: 2

Cooking Time: 0 Minutes

Ingredients:

- 1 peach
- 4 Mozzarella balls, cherry size
- ½ teaspoon pistachio, chopped
- 1 teaspoon honey

Directions:

1. Cut the peach on 4 cubes.

2. Then skewer peach cubes and Mozzarella balls on the skewers.

3. Sprinkle them with honey and chopped pistachio.

Nutrition Info:Per Serving:calories 202, fat 14.3, fiber 1.2, carbs 10, protein 10.8

Notes